BASAL CELL CARCINOMA

Finding Your Way Through Diagnosis, Treatment, and Beyond: The Chronicles of Basal Cell Carcinoma

JACE COOPER

Table of Contents

Introductory

Cancer of the skin known as basal cell carcinoma (BCC) begins in the basal cells of the epidermis, the skin's outermost layer. As older skin cells die off, they are replaced by new ones produced by basal cells. Long-term exposure to ultraviolet (UV) radiation from the sun or tanning beds is the leading cause of basal cell carcinoma (BCC), the most prevalent form of skin cancer.

• This malignancy tends to progress slowly and almost never spreads to other parts of the body, a phenomenon known as "metastasis." However, if untreated, it can spread to neighboring tissues, resulting in scarring. Pearly or waxy bumps on the skin, often with visible blood vessels; flat, flesh-colored or brown scar-like lesions are all possible presentations of basal cell carcinoma.

Successful management requires prompt diagnosis and treatment of basal cell carcinoma. Surgical excision, radiation therapy, and topical therapies may all be viable alternatives, depending on the nature and location of the tumor. BCC can be prevented and detected early by taking precautions against sun damage and keeping a close eye on the skin for any signs of change.

CHAPTER ONE
Reasons and Potential Threats

Basal cell carcinoma (BCC) is almost often caused by overexposure to UV rays, either from the sun or tanning beds. This exposure affects the DNA in skin cells, leading to mutations that can result in the development of cancer. But there are a few things that can raise a person's chance of getting BCC:

1. Prolonged and accumulated exposure to the sun, especially its harmful UV rays, is a significant risk factor for basal cell carcinoma (BCC). Those who spend a lot of time outside are more vulnerable, especially if they don't take precautions like wearing sunscreen or protective gear.

2. Indoor tanning with lamps or beds has been linked to an increased risk of skin cancer, particularly basal cell carcinoma. The UV radiation emitted by these devices is often more powerful than that of the sun.

3. People with fair skin have less melanin, making them less susceptible to the damaging effects of the sun's rays. As a result, they are more prone to skin damage and skin cancer.

4. A history of severe sunburns, especially in infancy, has been linked to an increased likelihood of acquiring BCC in adulthood. Burns are an indication of severe sun exposure to the skin.

5. A higher incidence of skin cancer has been linked to living in sunny, high-altitude places with high quantities of ultraviolet light.

6. One of the risk factors for developing BCC is a family history of the disease. The onset of skin cancer may have hereditary components.

7. A weakened immune system can raise the risk of skin cancer because it does not provide as much protection against the formation of malignant cells as a healthy one would.

8. Arsenic Exposure: Arsenic is present in certain well water and in some industrial settings, and long-term exposure to high amounts of arsenic is linked to an elevated risk of skin cancer.

9. In general, adults over the age of 50 have the highest incidence of basal cell carcinoma.

10. Gender: Men are at higher risk for developing BCC than women are, though the gender difference is closing.

Although these characteristics may enhance the likelihood of developing basal cell carcinoma, it is crucial to remember that people of all skin tones and ethnicities are susceptible to this disease. Protecting your skin from the sun, keeping an eye out for any changes in your skin, and being cautious when spending time outside in the sun are the best ways to lower your risk of basal cell carcinoma. Consult a healthcare provider or dermatologist if you have any concerns or risk factors about skin cancer.

Genetics and Vulnerability of the Skin

When it comes to skin cancers like basal cell carcinoma (BCC), an individual's skin type might play a major impact in their risk. Different varieties of skin are typically categorized according to how they react to the sun and other environmental factors. The Fitzpatrick scale is commonly used to classify skin types such as these:

1. People with skin type I (extremely fair) are naturally pale, and their skin burns easily in the sun. They are the most susceptible to sunburn and skin cancer.

2. People with Type II (Fair) skin are more prone to sunburn and develop only a little tan. They are also more susceptible to sunburn and skin cancer.

3. People with skin type III (light to medium) tend to have fair to medium skin that burns easily but eventually develops a tan. They run a lower than average risk of sunburn.

4. People with skin of Type IV (Olive) pigmentation rarely get sunburned and tan readily. They are less likely to become sunburned or suffer other skin problems.

5. People with skin type V (Brown) have naturally dark complexions that tan easily and sunburn very rarely. They aren't as likely to become sunburned.

6. Skin of Type VI (Very Dark) persons is naturally very dark, does not sunburn readily, and tans well. They are at the lowest risk for sunburn and skin damage.

These skin types may differ in their susceptibility to developing basal cell carcinoma and other forms of skin cancer. People with light skin (Types I and II) are especially vulnerable to sun damage because they have less melanin, the pigment in skin responsible for blocking UV light. The higher melanin content of those with darker skin tones (Types IV to VI) makes them less susceptible to sunburn and skin cancer.

To be clear, however, the effects of ultraviolet (UV) radiation can be felt by everyone, regardless of skin tone. Excessive exposure to the sun or UV radiation over time can cause skin cancer in anyone, regardless of skin tone.

The need of prevention and early detection is universal, regardless of skin color. Sunscreen, long sleeves, and a hat are all good places to start, but you should also seek out shade, avoid indoor tanning, and perform self-exams and visits to the dermatologist frequently to keep an eye out for any changes in your skin. It is important for people of all skin types to take precautions against sun damage and seek treatment for any signs of skin cancer as soon as possible.

CHAPTER TWO
Symptoms and Indicators

Basal cell carcinoma (BCC) commonly appears with specific signs and symptoms. Early detection and treatment are crucial in successfully controlling this type of skin cancer; therefore it's important to be aware of these symptoms. Symptoms of basal cell carcinoma (BCC) often include:

• Small, pearly, or waxy lump on the skin is a common symptom of basal cell carcinoma (BCC). This protrusion could be glossy, see-through, or glassy in appearance. It can be quite large later on, but normally starts off quite little.

• Visible, fine blood vessels running through the bump may give it a spidery or lacey appearance.

• Some BCCs progress into an open sore that doesn't heal, sometimes known as an ulcer. Occasionally, the wound may leak, crust over, or bleed.

• In some circumstances, basal cell carcinoma (BCC) can look like a faint scar on the skin. Possible skin depressions and a level surface.

• A pink or red area on the skin, which may be slightly elevated or scaly, is another symptom of basal cell carcinoma. This area may grow in size gradually.

• A glossy lump with a rolling, elevated border is a possible indicator of basal cell carcinoma. One comparison could be to an in-skin pearl.

• Mild Pain, discomfort, or itching in the afflicted area is a common symptom of BCC lesions.

• Any new, odd growth on the skin needs to be watched carefully. Concerns should be raised if a growth suddenly changes in size, form, color, or texture.

- BCC generally expands at a sluggish rate. It's vital to notice even small shifts because it could not alter significantly over several months.

Keep in mind that these symptoms may present differently in different people and might differ by BCC subtype. The face, ears, neck, scalp, chest, and back are common places to find basal cell carcinomas (BCCs), but they can appear anywhere on the body.

It is critical to see a doctor or dermatologist if you experience any changes to your skin, especially if they continue or are uncommon in nature. The likelihood of successfully controlling basal cell carcinoma and limiting its spread or inflicting more damage increases with earlier identification and therapy. The early stages of skin cancer and other skin abnormalities can be detected with regular self-examinations and expert skin inspections.

Diagnosis

A doctor, generally a dermatologist, will examine the suspicious mole to determine if it is basal cell carcinoma (BCC). The following may all be part of the diagnostic procedure for basal cell carcinoma:

- **Clinical Examination:** A healthcare expert, usually a dermatologist, may visually evaluate the skin for any unusual or abnormal growths, discolorations, or blemishes. They will take detailed notes on the skin anomaly, including its size, shape, color, and texture.

- Your healthcare professional may inquire about your medical history, which may include past skin disorders and/or skin cancer.

- The use of a dermatoscope is appropriate in specific situations. This handheld instrument facilitates a closer inspection of the skin lesion by the dermatologist. Certain characteristics of the lesion can be shown, which may assist determine if it is malignant or not.

• A skin biopsy may be recommended by the dermatologist if they have any doubts about the diagnosis of the skin lesion. A biopsy entails the removal of a tiny piece of the suspect tissue for further analysis in a lab. Several distinct forms of skin biopsies exist, including:

With a shave biopsy, only the top layer of the lesion is removed.

The lesion is eliminated by punching out a little, cylinder-shaped section of tissue.

• Incisional biopsy involves removing a small piece of the lesion for testing.

• Complete removal of the lesion (excisional biopsy).

The size and location of the lesion will determine which biopsy technique is most appropriate.

• Histopathological analysis occurs when a pathologist looks at the biopsy tissue under a microscope in a pathology lab. They will examine the tissue to see if it is cancerous and, if so, what kind of cancer it is and what features it displays.

• If a biopsy confirms basal cell carcinoma, additional testing may be required to ascertain the cancer's stage and whether or not it has spread. This may include imaging tests such as ultrasound, MRI, or CT scans, especially if the BCC is large or in a sensitive location.

Keep in mind that basal cell carcinoma (BCC) is typically a slow-growing, localized disease that seldom spreads to other sections of the body. Therefore, BCC may not always require the rigorous staging and tests used for other cancers. However, knowing the extent of the BCC is useful for planning treatment.

Effective management of basal cell carcinoma requires both early detection and rapid treatment. Important medical attention and consultation with a healthcare practitioner should be sought out in the event of any odd or persistent changes to the skin.

CHAPTER THREE
Categories and Subtypes

There are many subsets of basal cell carcinoma (BCC), each with its own set of symptoms and physical hallmarks. Understanding these classifications is crucial since they influence both treatment options and prognoses. Some typical forms of BCC are listed below:

• Most basal cell carcinomas are of the nodular variety. It often takes the form of a pearly or waxy lump on the skin with visible tiny blood vessels. It frequently ulcerates, resulting in a central sore.

- Superficial basal cell carcinoma looks like a red, scaly spot on the skin, like eczema or psoriasis. It spreads slowly and is most frequently seen on the trunk and limbs of a tree.

- The subtype of basal cell carcinoma known as morpheaform (sclerosing) BCC is known to be more aggressive and invasive than other types. It generally resembles a scar, with a white or yellowish tint and blurry edges. It can be difficult to spot, and removal might necessitate specialized procedures like Mohs surgery.

• Pigmented basal cell carcinoma (BCC): This type of BCC can be brown or black in color, like a melanoma. The similarity in hue to other skin disorders, such as benign moles or melanoma, can make diagnosis difficult.

• Pinkus fibroepithelioma is a kind of fibroepithelioma that typically manifests as a flesh-colored tumor on the lower back. This kind of BCC develops slowly and poses little threat overall.

• This kind of BCC, known as infundibulocystic BCC, develops in hair follicles and typically shows up as a cystic or nodular lesion on the head or trunk.

• This subtype of BCC, known as adenosquamous (basosquamous), can have characteristics with both basal cell carcinoma and squamous cell carcinoma. It tends to be more severe and may necessitate expert care.

• The head and neck are prominent locations for keratotic (desmoplastic) BCC, which is characterized by a thick, fibrous tissue architecture. It can be difficult to treat and might cause localized damage.

• Infiltrative basal cell carcinoma: Basal cell carcinomas with indistinct borders tend to infect neighboring tissues more vigorously. It usually takes the form of a smooth scar.

• Sometimes basal cell carcinoma will form several lesions in the same geographic region, a condition known as multifocal or multicentric BCC. This can make it more difficult to diagnose and plan therapy.

It's crucial to note that while some BCC subtypes are less aggressive and slow-growing, others might be more invasive and challenging to treat. All subtypes of basal cell carcinoma (BCC) require prompt detection and treatment. If you observe any suspicious skin changes or growths, it's crucial to visit a dermatologist for a proper evaluation and diagnosis, since the choice of therapy may depend on the individual type of BCC and its characteristics.

Choices in Medical Care

Basal cell carcinoma (BCC) can be treated in a number of different ways. BCC therapy options are condition- and patient-specific, taking into account the specifics of the patient's diagnosis and stage of disease. Common methods of dealing with BCC include:

1. Excision surgery is the most common and primary treatment for basal cell carcinoma. During excision, the malignant tissue is removed and the margins are checked to make sure they are cancer-free. After the tumor has been surgically removed, a sample of the excised tissue is submitted to a lab for further examination.

2. When a basal cell carcinoma (BCC) is particularly large, aggressive, or located in an aesthetically delicate location, a surgeon may opt for Mohs micrographic surgery, a specialized and highly accurate surgical method. Until no cancer cells are found, the surgeon carefully removes and examines tiny layers of tissue under a microscope. In order to reduce unnecessary tissue loss, Mohs surgery is often used.

3. The doctor uses a curette to scrape out the tumor, and then an electric needle to cauterize the region (electrodessication), in a process known as curettage and electrodessication. The procedure can be repeated as needed for smaller, more clearly defined BCCs.

4. Radiation therapy is an alternative to surgical removal for individuals with advanced disease, those with particular medical issues, or those who have lesions in aesthetically sensitive locations. High-energy X-rays are focused on the tumor in an effort to eradicate cancer cells.

5. Freezing, or cryotherapy, involves exposing the tumor to liquid nitrogen in order to kill cancer cells. Small, superficial BCCs are the usual candidates for this treatment.

6. Some BCCs, particularly the superficial forms, respond well to prescription topical lotions or gels. Imicumod and 5-fluorouracil (5-FU) are two such examples. These drugs work by boosting the immune system's ability to recognize and destroy cancer cells.

7. Treatment with a laser, which emits a concentrated beam of light, can obliterate the BCC. As a rule, it is reserved for superficial or minor BCCs.

8. In photodynamic therapy (PDT), a photosensitizing drug is first applied to the tumor before it is exposed to a narrow spectrum of light. This triggers the agent's ability to kill cancer cells selectively. In some cases of superficial BCCs, it is used.

9. Oral medicines such as vismodegib and sonidegib have been approved for the treatment of advanced BCCs or BCCs that cannot be cured with surgery or radiation. The growth of BCCs is inhibited because they attack the molecular pathways responsible for this.

The specifics of the BCC, its location, the patient's general health, and the patient's preferences all play a role in determining the best course of therapy. Early diagnosis and therapy are critical for optimal management of BCC. The best course of therapy depends on your individual circumstances, therefore it's best to talk to a doctor or dermatologist about it. The best way to prevent a recurrence and make sure everything works out is to schedule regular follow-up appointments.

CHAPTER FOUR
Recuperation and Follow-Up

Recuperation and follow-up care are crucial stages in the management of basal cell carcinoma (BCC). Depending on the nature of your treatment and your current health, the time it takes and the specific processes involved in your recovery may differ. Some broad principles and factors to think about during recuperation and follow-up care are outlined below.

• Obey Your Doctor's Orders your doctor's orders and recommendations for post-treatment care should be strictly adhered to. This may involve following a prescribed drug schedule, maintaining a sanitary wound site, or using a special skincare regimen.

• **Care for a Wound:** After BCC removal surgery, you may have a wound that needs specific attention. Always change your dressings as your doctor instructs you to, and make sure the affected area stays clean and dry.

• **Pain Relief:** You may feel some pain or discomfort as a result of your therapy, but how bad it is will vary from person to person and treatment to treatment. If you're experiencing pain, your doctor can prescribe medicine or suggest over-the-counter alternatives.

• Keep the treated area out of direct sunlight while it's healing. Sunscreen and other skin protection measures should be maintained even after skin cancer has been treated and the patient is feeling better.

• Appointments to check in on your progress and look for recurrence will be scheduled at regular intervals by your healthcare provider. These follow-up sessions are needed to ensure the malignancy is totally removed.

• **Cosmetic Considerations:** Depending on the location and size of the treated region, you may have cosmetic issues. Consult your doctor about possible treatments to lessen the appearance of scars or enhance the condition of the damaged skin.

• It is essential to take proper care of your skin after receiving therapy. To avoid drying out your skin, apply a mild moisturizer without any added scent. Don't use anything on your skin that might be too harsh or unpleasant in case it irritates the treated region.

• Modify your way of life if you need to in order to lower your risk of developing skin cancer. To do this, you should stay out of tanning beds, always use sunscreen and protective clothes, and seek shade during the hottest parts of the day.

• Check for new or changing skin lesions by doing self-examinations on a consistent basis. It's crucial to catch any unusual shifts early on in order to stop them from happening again.

• Learn the significance of early detection and skin protection. Learn about the causes and remedies for skin cancer.

In most cases, patients undergoing treatment for BCC make a full recovery and return to their pre-treatment levels of functioning within a short period of time. The prognosis for BCC is usually extremely excellent, especially with early discovery and effective treatment. But it's important to keep an eye out for any signs of a recurrence or new skin lesions, so it's important to continue taking precautions like staying out of the sun and getting frequent skin checks. Talk to your doctor or dermatologist if you have any concerns or questions about your treatment and subsequent care.

Recuperation and Follow-Up

Basal cell carcinoma (BCC) patients have a lot riding on their ability to recover and take care of themselves after undergoing therapy. The particular steps and duration of recovery can vary based on the sort of treatment you had and your individual health. Some broad principles and factors to think about during recuperation and follow-up care are outlined below.

• It is essential that you carefully adhere to your doctor's post-treatment care instructions. To do so, you may need to follow instructions for taking medications, treating wounds, and caring for your skin.

• The treatment of a wound may be necessary if a surgical or other procedure was used to remove the BCC. Follow your doctor's directions for cleaning, dressing changes, and maintaining the region free from infection.

• Intensity of discomfort or pain may vary from person to person and from treatment to treatment. If you're experiencing pain, your doctor can prescribe medicine or suggest over-the-counter alternatives.

• Avoid getting the treated area or any of your skin exposed to direct sunlight. Wear long-sleeved shirts and hats with a brim, as well as sunscreen with an SPF of at least 30. Stay out of tanning beds and midday sun.

• Appointments to check in on your progress and look for recurrence will be scheduled at regular intervals by your healthcare provider. These checkups are crucial for ensuring total cancer eradication and addressing any questions or concerns you may have.

• **Cosmetic Considerations:** Depending on the location and size of the treated region, you may have cosmetic issues. Consult your doctor about treatments that can lessen the appearance of scars or restore the skin's normal texture and tone.

• It is essential to take proper care of your skin after receiving therapy. Moisturize frequently using a mild, fragrance-free product to avoid skin dryness and irritation. Don't use anything that could irritate your skin.

- **Modifying Your Way of Life:** Altering your way of life may help minimize your risk of developing skin cancer. If you must be outside during high sun hours, it is best to protect yourself by staying indoors, wearing protective clothing, sunglasses, and sunscreen.

- **Self-Skin Exams:** You should keep up with your routine self-skin checks to detect any new or changing skin lesions. The key to preventing a recurrence is prompt notice of any worrisome changes.

• Learn as much as you can about the causes and preventative measures for skin cancer. Learn more about skin protection and early detection and how they can help you.

In most cases, patients undergoing treatment for BCC make a full recovery and return to their pre-treatment levels of functioning within a short period of time. The prognosis for BCC is usually extremely excellent, especially with early discovery and effective treatment. But it's important to keep an eye out for any signs of a recurrence or new skin lesions, so it's important to wear sunscreen and examine your skin regularly.

Talk to your doctor or dermatologist if you have any concerns or questions about your treatment and subsequent care. Based on the details of your case, they can provide you the best recommendations.

CHAPTER FIVE
Making Peace with the Prognosis

Although learning that you have basal cell carcinoma (BCC) may be upsetting, there are ways to deal with the news and overcome potential obstacles. Some ways to deal with hearing that you have BCC are listed below.

• Get informed about basal cell carcinoma (BCC), its causes, risk factors, and available treatments. Fear and worry might be reduced by learning as much as you can about your situation.

• **Seek out Support:** Tell trusted friends and family members so they can help you cope with the news. Having someone you can lean on during diagnosis and treatment can be a huge help.

• It is essential that you provide complete and frank information with your healthcare team. Ask questions regarding the diagnosis, treatment choices, and expected outcomes. The professionals caring for you can provide you advice and answer your questions.

• Feelings like fear, worry, grief, and rage are all natural responses that must be managed. Let yourself feel what you're feeling, and if you need to, go to a counselor or other mental health expert.

• Consider participating in a support group for those who have been diagnosed with skin cancer or BCC. Having access to a community of people who have overcome comparable obstacles can be a great source of both emotional and intellectual support.

• Maintain Knowledge of Your Treatment: Know What Your Doctor Suggested. Feeling more in charge of your circumstances is possible when you know what to anticipate during treatment.

• Despite the fact that learning you have BCC can be upsetting, it is usually quite curable, especially if caught early. Focus on the possibility of making a full recovery, and maintain an optimistic mindset.

• In order to prevent further skin damage and limit the risk of developing skin malignancies, it is important to continue to protect your skin from sun exposure even while undergoing treatment and recuperation.

• Adherence to the treatment plan is crucial to achieving the desired results. Always follow your doctor's orders and take your prescription.

• If you are having a hard time processing your emotions after receiving a diagnosis, you may benefit from talking to a trained professional.

• Eat well, move often, and get enough of shut-eye to keep your body in tip-top shape. A healthy lifestyle can support your general well-being during and after treatment.

• Take time for yourself and do things that make you happy and relaxed. Activities like yoga, meditation, and spending time with loved ones all fit into this category.

- Although it's crucial to stay educated, it's also important to avoid over-researching your health online, as doing so might cause undue concern. Stick to trusted sources for information.

Keep in mind that basal cell carcinoma is an extremely curable, slow-growing kind of skin cancer. The prognosis can be improved with early diagnosis and the right therapy. By actively managing your health, getting assistance, and concentrating on your general well-being, you can better manage with the diagnosis and the problems it provides.

Conclusion

The most prevalent type of skin cancer is called basal cell carcinoma (BCC), and it is caused by overexposure to the sun or tanning beds. Early detection and treatment are crucial for the successful management of BCC, despite the fact that it grows slowly and seldom spreads to other parts of the body.

• The key to early detection and prevention of BCC is knowledge of the disease's symptoms, risk factors, and subtypes. Seeking medical assistance quickly is essential if you notice any suspicious changes in your skin.

• Depending on the nature of the tumor and its location, BCC can be treated in a number of ways, including through surgery, radiation therapy, topical medicines, and other specialist approaches. Proper wound care, sun protection, routine follow-up checkups, and periodic self-skin checks are all essential parts of recovery and aftercare following treatment.

• Individuals can successfully manage the disease and focus on preserving their overall well-being with the help of healthcare professionals, friends, and family, as well as by remaining knowledgeable and positive.

In all facets of dealing with BCC, from prevention to diagnosis, treatment, and recovery, remaining aware and proactive is crucial to ensure the best possible outcome. Prevention of skin cancer and early detection of skin cancer through frequent skin checks are crucial for a higher likelihood of a successful recovery and sustained health.

THE END